36 Days Apart

*A Memoir of a daughter, her parents and the Beast
named – Alzheimer's
A story of Life, Love and Death*

Deborah Ann Tornillo

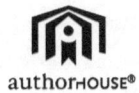

authorHOUSE®

AuthorHouse™
1663 Liberty Drive
Bloomington, IN 47403
www.authorhouse.com
Phone: 1-800-839-8640

First published by AuthorHouse 4/15/2009

ISBN: 978-1-4389-5233-8 (sc)

Library of Congress Control Number: 2009903607

Printed in the United States of America
Bloomington, Indiana

This book is printed on acid-free paper.

Prologue

In Your Honor

Death has taken you from this world, and though we are apart, you
are still near.
All that we meant to each other remains true, in trust and faith,
have no fear.

I'll keep you always close to my heart, for you left me what no one
can steal,
a treasure chest of precious, happy memories: the tender love-filled
moments we shared, as well as the challenging times that brought
us closer together.

When I'm in need, I'll speak to you, and call your name.
You will come to me with wisdom and light, to fill my soul with
peace,
and to guide me in the pathways that lead to life forever with our
Loving God.

Your sacred promise to me, when you are home in God's embrace,
is whenever I call,
you will still be present to me, for neither death nor grave can break
the bonds of love that we on earth once knew.

You will be missed, but never forgotten!

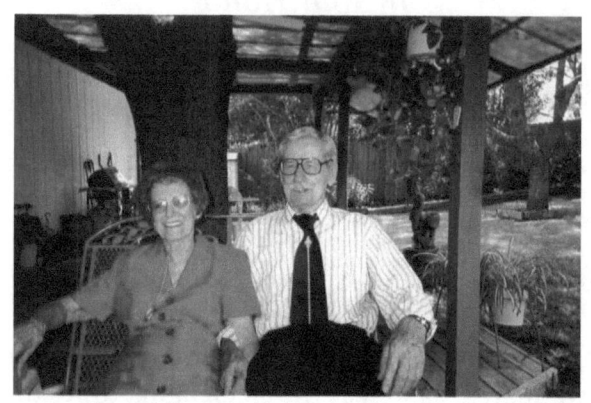

Acknowledgement

Thank you family and friends (you know who you are) for all your support during the process of taking care of Mom and Dad. I couldn't have done it without you and will always be grateful for you in my life. Thank you God for when I felt alone and not able to carry on, you lifted my spirit and gave me the strength and courage I needed.

I love you Mom and Dad and always will and thank you for trusting in me to care of you. My last gift to you is to share the story of your life, your love and your death with generations to come.

Introduction

I didn't know when I would tell this story, I just knew I would. Both my mother and father had Alzheimer's; my Mom was further along in the disease process than my Dad. It was an incredible journey spending the last year and a half of their life with them, slowly watching the disease take its toll. Alzheimer's is a living death and although I have witnessed first hand this dreadful disease in both parents, I have been blessed to have been by their side throughout this journey and hold their hand as far as I could.

The two most important things I learned from my parents as we traveled this road together was how to stay strong in faith and never lose compassion for others or myself. I was blessed to have learned from them their wisdom of life and death.

I have faith that as you read my parent's story you will gain the strength and wisdom needed to guide you.

February, 2006

I remember as if it were yesterday, when the telephone rang and it was my sister, Sue. She told me while on her visit each Sunday to see Mom and Dad, that things just didn't seem right with them. She lived in Texas, approximately a thirty minute drive from them, while I was in Virginia. She would visit them every Sunday and started noticing little things at first, regarding their activities of daily living. The house seemed messier than usual, there was never any food in the refrigerator, and their appearance was being neglected. The biggest change she noticed was in my mother. She would express her concern to me that Mom just seemed to be losing it mentally. I could hear the fear in Sue's voice. I knew then that it was time that I travel to Texas to check things out for myself, because my parents were always so organized, meticulous and I couldn't comprehend them ever being any other way.

The morning I boarded the plane there was an air of excitement within me for I was returning to Texas to see Mom and Dad. I was also looking forward to spending time with my sister and my daughter, Courtney. As I sat in my cramped seat on the airplane, I found myself thinking not about my present journey, but about the time my sister came to visit me in Virginia, Christmas of 2002. It was a very difficult time for Sue, because Mom had been accusing her of stealing things out of their home and Sue was so devastated by my mother's accusations.

Apparently, these accusations had been going on for months and I could not understand what was going on with Mom, nor could I ever imagine where all of this would take me.

I started thinking about how Mom no longer emailed me. She had convinced Dad many years ago to buy her a computer and she spent endless hours each day emailing everyone. She was great at emailing me to catch up on the latest, but as the years went by I noticed the emails stopped coming. When I would confront her about it she would simply say she did reply to my email, or made some excuse about her computer not working.

During that same Christmas Day, the phone rang here at my home in Virginia and it was Mom. She sounded wonderful and wished me a Merry Christmas. She then asked to speak to Sue, at which time she apologized to her. The tears of joy flooded my sister's eyes. I was so happy that on this joyous day of the year, they had come to peace. What I did not know at the time, was Dad had made up some story to Mom that a burglar had come in to their house and stole whatever she was claiming was missing. I then spoke with Dad and wished him a Merry Christmas and his reply back was "Blah Humbug". He always could bring a smile to me. Thanks to Dad he once again saved the day!

As I continued to reminisce on the flight I thought about how many things had changed. I rarely received phone calls from Mom or Dad and found myself always calling them. Every time I would call, Dad would answer the phone, tell me he's doing fine, ask me how the family was doing and then call Mom to the phone. I had also noticed when I would talk with Mom how often she would repeat a story to me that she had previously told me. I didn't give it much thought and just attributed it to old age.

When I arrived at their home I was greeted with lots of hugs and kisses. I noticed that they both appeared thinner, but yet looked okay.

It felt so good to be with Mom and Dad. We started catching up on good and bad times with the family, of course with me doing all the talking and them just listening. When it was time for lunch Mom offered me a chicken patty sandwich, which was one of her favorites. After lunch, Dad quickly rose from the table to clean the dishes. I thought how amazing it was that their routine never seemed to change. As he moved around the kitchen I sensed a weakness in him that I had never sensed before. I had asked him if he was okay, and just like Dad's typical Dad answer – Yes, I'm fine! He then excused himself to his TV room which he called "The Hooch". There he remained the rest of the afternoon watching his programs, but sleeping most of the time. Occasionally on my trip to the restroom, I would pass his room and peek in at him and remind myself that he was my rock, so content with himself, so strong, and always so positive. Yet, I had a deep feeling inside of me that something was wrong.

While Dad watched TV and slept Mom and I spent the remainder of the afternoon gossiping and her repeating her many stories she had previously told me. There was an obsession about her regarding burglars breaking into their house and stealing all of her jewelry. She would show me where she had now hidden her remaining jewelry and would talk over and over about all the other pieces that were stolen. I was thrilled that afternoon to leave their house and go spend the night at my sisters. I couldn't wait to get away from what seemed in the few hours that I was there a very depressing energy in my parent's house. Sue and I had a great evening catching up. She and I have always been close and as I listened to her concerns regarding Mom and Dad I knew deep down inside of me that something wasn't right and I felt major changes were coming, what those changes would be I did not know.

The next day, my sister went to work and I drove over to see Mom and Dad. I arrived around 9:30 and they were still at the kitchen table

3

having their breakfast and reading the newspaper. I thought how nice it was to be retired with no schedule constraints, just take your time and do as you please. I watched as Dad started his routine of feeding Silky their cat and Poncho their dog, clean the kitchen and then clean the litter box. I noticed the effort it took him to do this. I noticed the deep breathing coming from him for such a little bit of effort. At one point when he stood, he became very dizzy, but just quickly said it was no big deal. I asked him if he was okay and he simply said he was fine. I noticed how Mom continued to have the same conversation about the robbers coming into their house as if she was telling me for the very first time. I noticed as Dad washed the breakfast dishes he used only water and no soap.

I noticed after his morning chores he excused himself to The Hooch to watch his favorite program "Wheel of Fortune". I noticed while passing The Hooch, on the way to the restroom he was sleeping. I noticed in the restroom, how dirty the floors were. I noticed the scotch tape on the locks of the doors. I noticed the nails in the windows to prevent them from being opened. I noticed the 2 by 4 piece of wood in their bedroom that was used to prop up against their door so the robbers could not get in. I noticed them both wearing the same thing they had on the day before. They needed my help, but yet how was I going to help them living so far away.

"Dear God, guide me on how to take care of my parents who have taken care of me their whole life." "I'm afraid."

That afternoon, I made the decision to stay at their house the night and just observe the rest of the day and evening. I spent the remainder of the afternoon with Mom watching TV, while Dad sat in "The Hooch" watching TV, or should I say sleeping. Mom's favorite program was Meerkat Manor and what I did not realize at the time that this was her only program that she remembered how to get to. I would tell her to

4

change the channel to something else and she would tell me that there was nothing else on. I accommodated her, because I was just simply there to observe. That evening, I prepared supper. They both ate very well. I also surprised them with a wonderful chocolate cake for dessert. They were very thankful for the meal. After supper, Dad started his routine of cleaning the kitchen, but this time I immediately took over to make sure the dishes were cleaned properly. Mom would try to do her part, but she just mostly got in the way, as if she was disoriented as to what to do. It was after this meal that I noticed Mom asking Dad if the dog and cat had eaten. Yes, he would say to her in his calm voice. Three minutes later, she would ask the question again. I found myself almost becoming irritated at her. I still hadn't connected all the dots.

That evening, my father joined us to watch TV. After our big bowls of chocolate ice cream mother excused herself for bedtime. I watched her walkover to the front door of our house, and check the locks and then she took coat hanger wire that was on the floor and started to wrap it all around the door handle. She then took my grandmother's trunk and pushed it in front of the door. She then went into the utility room and made sure that door which lead to the garage was just as secured with scotch tape. She then came over to me and gave me a kiss and went into her bedroom. I was shocked by her actions. I didn't know what to say. I turned to Dad and he looked at me and said "she does that every night and if it makes her feel safe, then no big deal." I thought to myself "safe, safe from what"? Dad and I enjoyed the remainder of the evening watching TV. Sitting with him made me feel safe and I could not understand why Mom didn't feel the same. As I lay in bed that night millions of thoughts entered my head. Where do I start, what do I do? Will they let me take care of them? Will I be intruding? I did not want to take away their independence, but yet in the two short days that I observed them, they definitely needed help.

The next morning, Dad drove himself to the bank. Every month, the first Monday of the month he would drive himself to the bank to get cash. Every week, the first Monday of each week Dad also did all the grocery shopping. And, it became apparent as the days went on that he did the cleaning. When I would approach my Dad about this, he would simply say "no big deal". My father use to always say that to me. He would turn to me in his strong, fatherly voice and say to me "don't make a big deal about it Debbie". My father the rock!

After a week long visit, I left Mom and Dad. I left knowing that I would return soon and knew that when I got home to Virginia that I needed to start researching as much as I could about Alzheimer and Dementia, because my gut feeling was they had the disease. I researched on how to take over their financial affairs and how to do it without offending them. I researched on finding someone to take care of them and their daily activities of living, while respecting their independence. But, what I was not able to research, was how to present all these necessary changes to my Dad, without him feeling loss of dignity, respect and most important in his mind – his strength as a man. Although I was afraid of what the future held, I knew deep down inside of me that I had to take care of them and by the grace of God he would guide me.

March, 2006

When I arrived home to Virginia I was overwhelmed with a flood of thoughts of where to begin. I knew I needed to gather as much information in as short of a period of time that I possibly could, because I needed to return to Texas as soon as I could. I still felt confident that Dad was capable of taking care of things until I returned, but yet my gut told me not for long.

Thanks to the Internet I had a wealth of information in front of me on the subject of Alzheimer. I knew that even though I had formulated a plan, that there would be continuous tweaking as we went through it. I also prayed daily to God to help guide me through each day to be the best that I could be in order to help my parents with their daily activities of living. There are literally hundreds of terrific websites on the internet that also helped me through this journey and these are just a few of them that I used to help formulate my plan of the things that I needed to do in order to get started:

http://www.alz.org/
http://www.eldercare.gov/Eldercare/Public/Home.asp
http://www.aarp.org/families/caregiving/
http://www.eldercarelink.com/
http://www.caringinfo.org/

http://www.caringinfo.org/UserFiles/File/
PDFs/AdvanceCarePlanningLegalIssues/
AGuideToLegalIssuesInLifeLimitingConditions.pdf
www.nhpco.org

MY LIST

Assessing Their Needs:
- Do they need help with grooming, bathing, or dressing?
- Do they need help with housekeeping, shopping, or yard work?
- Do they need help with meal planning and preparation?
- Do they need help with transportation?
- Do they need help making legal and other important decisions?
- Do they have trouble functioning at home? Would modifications help?
- Do they have any physical limitations with hearing, vision, or memory?

Getting Their Permission:
- Durable Power of Attorney to make legal decisions
- Medical Power of Attorney to make health care decisions

Access to Personal & Financial Information:
- Insurance (Medicare / Medicaid numbers, supplements, other policies)
- Doctors names, phone numbers and other contact information
- Medical history of medications, allergies, conditions, procedures

- Identification (social security, military ID, Drive License numbers)
- Address List of friends, neighbors and family
- Service Providers (Attorney, financial advisor, clergy, accountant)
- Financial account numbers, checkbook, investments, tax records
- Legal (Wills, Power of Attorney, Health Care Directive)
- Original documents (house, other property, car title)
- Insurance (Life, medical, auto, homeowners)
- Vital Records (Original birth certificates, marriage license, military records)

Having a heart to heart conversation with them:
- Their personal wishes (finances, medical treatments, funeral, burial, organ donation and their property distribution.

Important Care giving Responsibilities:
- Respect their independence
- Allow them to make as many decisions as appropriate
- Keep reasonable expectations of what they can do independently
- Talk regularly with them about their concerns, desires, and frustrations
- Make informed decisions that are in the best interest of your parent's needs
- Show compassion while you are trying to be efficient and responsible

Take Care of Yourself:
- Recognize when you are worn out and need a break

April, 2006

This time as I sat on a plane returning to Texas I was happy that I was returning with a plan. I had also prepared copies of the Texas Statutory Durable Power of Attorney and Medical Power of Attorney Designation of Health Care Agent for both of my parents' signature. I questioned how they would respond to me returning with these documents, basically asking them to sign over all their affairs to me and my sister.

I knew in my heart that my mother would show concern for all of this, because at this point I was convinced she had Alzheimer. I just didn't know what stage of the disease she was in and planned to investigate that further, but first things first was to put a safety net in place for them.

Mom and Dad greeted me at the door with lots of hugs and kisses. It felt so good to be there and a peace fell over me knowing that now that I was there, they would be okay. My father was especially excited to see me. I sensed a big relief in him. With me there now, it was quite obvious he relaxed and was right back to his routine of sleeping in The Hooch. My concern was why he was sleeping so much. Again, I just attributed it to old age. I remember the many times I would talk to Mom on the telephone and how upset she would be with him. She would complain about how much time he spent in his Hooch sleeping. Mom was bored, living in that big house all by herself, no companionship other then when my Dad made his appearance every once in a while to sneak in a bit of candy. He had such a sweet tooth and I loved to surprise him with great desserts after dinner. On one of my grocery shopping trips I introduced him to Rocky Road Ice cream. That became the only ice cream he wanted to eat from that point on. The mornings would arrive and I would have already been up and out the door before they woke and would have waiting for him fresh out of the oven glazed donuts. He couldn't get enough of it and I realized as time went on he became more and more dependent on me. It was very soon into this visit that I explained to them about the Power of Attorney and Medical Power of Attorney forms that I had with me. I also discussed with them the need for having someone come into the house and help them with the activities of daily living. I was surprised that I did not get any resistance from Dad regarding the finances. He was ready to give that job to me in a heart beat. I had come to find out that he had been doing it a long time. My guess is since 2002 when my mother first started showing signs of Alzheimer. On this visit I went with Dad to the bank for his monthly visit. On our way to the bank that morning, he told me that he would take his statements each month into the bank and was having the bank's vice president reconcile his statement for him and he would also withdrawal $1000 worth of cash to get him by through the month. I questioned this process, but not to my Dad, for I respected whatever he did.

When we arrived at the bank we were greeted by Janet the vice president of the bank. She treated my father with such dignity and respect, but yet I could tell that she was extremely excited that I was there. It was from this day on that Janet and I formed a relationship that would help me with the process of caring for my parents finances. This was also the first sign that I saw in Dad that he didn't know what he was doing. He even admitted that to me and was so thankful to have Janet and that he wanted Janet and I to work together so I could take over all of his financial affairs. Several days later we completed the signing and witnessing of the Texas Statutory Durable Power of Attorney and Medical Power of Attorney Designation of Health Care Agent. It was also during this time that Janet had told me that she had been reconciling their bank statement for the past two years and also of some mistakes that could have cost my parents their whole savings. On one occasion my father had dropped his wallet inside the bank. On another occasion he had written a check to AOL for their monthly service and instead of it being $25.00, he wrote it for the balance of his checkbook, which was several thousand dollars. With this behind me, I knew the next thing that I needed to work on was convincing Dad that he need not carry so much cash on him. But respecting his independence, I would let it go until later. Dad loved to pass out cash and many times he gave Mom large sums to carry in her purse.

I remembered one visit in 2005 when I went to Wal-Mart with Mom and when it was time for her to pay she opened her wallet and pulled out all this money and put it on the counter. She was fumbling trying to make sense of all of it in order to give the cashier the right amount. As I look back on that time it is obvious now how she was struggling with the disease of Alzheimer. Dad would also pass out large sums of money to his grandchildren whenever they would visit. He was so generous.

With the banking formalities out of the way, I spent the next several weeks at their house going through all their personal files. They kept excellent records and I found all original documents and secured those to bring home with me to start trying to understand what was going on with their estate. When Dad took over the bank statement he managed to keep a handwritten log of everything. I was also fortunate to find on my mother's computer important information that she had stored. I found one particular document that was dated 2003 that had listed things that were missing in her home. Within this document she itemized things that were missing, but she also tried to list birthdates and death dates of relatives. I felt at the time she was just trying to remember things. God bless her.

During this visit I also managed to convince Dad that it would be in the best interest for Mom to bring in a home health aide to assist with her. I explained to Dad the importance of this because of the safety issues that could arise, and also it would allow him to rest. I knew that he had been trying to do it all for many years. The Home Health Agency sent me Sarah. She was to work a total of 5 hours per day. This was all that Dad would agree to. As his daughter I respected him. I left Texas and returned to Virginia feeling secure in what I had accomplished this trip. The safety net was in place for their finances and their well being.

May, 2006

The month of May was spent trying to get myself organized with all their files that I brought home with me. I knew that I had to learn as much as I could about where they stood financially, because of the high cost of Home Health Care, as well as just wrap my arms around their life up to this point. I spent hours, upon hours reading through each and every piece of paper. There were so many interesting things that I learned about my parents that I had never known before. It was wonderful going over original documents and thinking to myself what it must have been like for them when they first got married, bought their first house, gave birth to their first child. All the original documents were right before my eyes. I felt blessed to have been given the opportunity to ingest as much as I could, but more important to hold on to these important documents for generations to come.

My biggest challenge was to go through all the paperwork that Dad had kept from his services in the military. He proudly served our country with the 501st Paratrooper Infantry Regiment, Company D, and 101st Airborne Division in the U. S. Army during WWII, receiving a Purple Heart for injuries he sustained during combat. As I read through the personal journal that my father kept of his war days, I was enthralled over what a strong man he was then and even up to the final hours of his death. I feel honored and blessed that I was given the opportunity to share this part of my Dad's life.

Excerpts from Dad's Journal:

July 12, 1944 – "I dedicate this journal to the Men of my Platoon who cannot be here in England, because they died in France in the invasion, to let others continue life. **"WE SALUTE YOU"!**

July 13, 1944 "In England, after our return from the Normandy Invasion – it looks beautiful. Its rolling hills and peaceful countryside, minus the untold miseries of war – not as France, it to was once carefree and proud, now it is stripped of its glory and raped by our enemy. But someday soon she shall rise again among her fellow countries and again hold her head high. Viva La France!.

July 19, 1944 – How I wish this damn war was over.

August 3, 1944 – "The men are working and training strenuously – little sleep and recreation. They know what faces them in the very near future, another combat jump behind enemy lines to repay the fanatic murderers for the lives of their comrades who died so gallantly, some still in their chutes, others before they had a chance to jump from their planes. It's a hell of a way to die. Yet it is my belief for a just cause – the enemy paid triple our cost."

September 17, 1944 – "We dropped in Holland and immediately obtained our objective. As I stood in the door of my plane and flew over Belgium and into Holland, we met very little flak. We dropped on our D.Z. and did not lose a single man. We captured a small town. My platoon was the first to reach it – the Holland people nearly went mad with joy. They gave us beer, wine, tea, cake, sandwiches and ice cream. They kissed and hugged us madly. In exchange, we gave them smokes, candy and silk from our parachutes."

September 23, 1944 – "We have just been attacked by the enemy – two of our tanks have been knocked out. The enemy lost one. The enemy's artillery and mortar barrage has been terrific – casualties in the company have been high." "Mom, your picture is right here in my book – that alone is my only inspiration to go on."

"Thousands of transports and gliders are now passing overhead. As I watch from my foxhole, I see transports being shot out of the sky – they don't stand a chance – flak is heavy in this area. Those boys have a lot of guts to fly those big, slow moving planes over here, but we are thankful for the supplies they are bringing."

September 27, 1944 – My radio operator and I were eating our rations when a shell hit beside us. It tore off his right arm and tore up his guts. It missed me completely. He was a damn good man, always by my side with his radio. I'm lost without him."

"It has been 11 days now since we jumped here. How I would like to be able to take off my boots and wash my feet or even shave my face.

September 30, 1944 – "Yes, I saw men of steal with tears in their eyes the day Sgt. Choate, my first squad sergeant was shot through the head. I told my best friend, Sgt. Koss of it, his best friend. There amidst all the hell and furious noise along the front lines of battle, I saw tears come to the eyes of the bearded young sergeant. I watched him break to pieces at the loss of his comrade."

"Life here has never told yet all its miseries"!

"Yesterday, I received a letter from the sister of a young corporal who was killed in action, but a second before the invasion of France had begun. He and 19 men were killed when their plane blew apart in mid-air. Cpl. Harris' sister wrote and asked if I could possibly tell her and her mother how her son was killed, and if I were really sure that he was dead. What more can I tell a Mother that has lost her son for the cause we are one and all fighting for. Should I tell her that he never had a chance to fight for *his life or that the corporal and 19 other men met their deaths in mid-air. ---- God, I hope this war ends very soon and that no more mothers have to suffer over the loss of their sons."*

As I read each day of Dad's journal I better understood what shaped this great man. It was the difficult times of war that shaped him. It was because of those difficult times of war that taught him life lessons. And it was because of war that gave him the strength that no father should have to endure, but the loss of his own son, my brother. Danny was killed in Vietnam and is still listed as KIA/BNR (Killed in Action/Body Not Recovered).

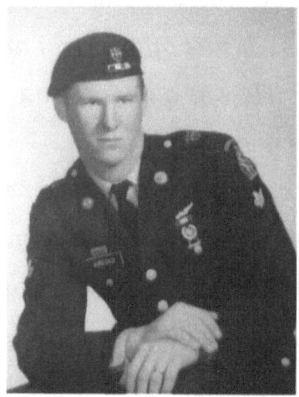

On May 8 1968, my brother and 3 other heroic men comprised the crew of a UH1C gunship in a flight of aircraft conducting a combat support mission against the NVA troops moving through the rugged jungle covered mountains of Vietnam. As the helicopter completed a turn from the east to the west members of other aircraft saw it explode in midair and plunge in flames into the bank of the Vuong River. The other flight members believed the violent midair explosion was the result of the Huey taking a direct hit from an explosive projectile.

Shortly after the incident, search and recovery (SAR) personnel were airlifted into the vicinity of the crash site, but due to enemy activity in the area, were only able to examine the wreckage from a distance. During their cursory examination, they found no signs of life in or around the crash site. Four days later, on May 12, 1968, a ground reconnaissance patrol from the 5th Special Forces Group was able to enter the crash site. They located the remains of the aircrew. Two of the charred bodies were found in the wreckage, the third along side of it and forth was 2 meters forward of the aircraft. All bodies were burned beyond recognition. Due to continued heavy enemy activity in the area and the badly deteriorated state of the remains, none of the bodies were recovered at that time and the search was terminated – and all 4 were immediately listed Killed in Action/Body Not Recovered.

I remembered, as I watched Mom and Dad in the days that followed the death of my brother I observed an undying faith and hope that someday my brother's body would be recovered and brought home for proper burial. That faith and hope is now seeded inside me. On October 7, 1944 Dad was wounded in combat and spent four and a half months in a hospital before making the long journey home by ship to America. He spoke in his journal about the long voyage home and five thousand wounded men on that ship. Some legless, armless, blind, deaf, shell shocked and what-not. Yet every man was happy because home lies ahead.

June, 2006

I returned to Texas for two very important reasons. One, to establish a Geriatric doctor for Mom and Dad and two, interview a new home health aide for them. I was successful at finding Mom and Dad a Geriatric doctor who evaluated both of them with Alzheimer's disease. He felt Mom was at the middle level of the disease and Dad was at the beginning.

Alzheimer's disease is a progressive neurological disease of the brain that leads to the irreversible loss of neurons and dementia. The clinical hallmarks of Alzheimer's disease are progressive impairment in memory, judgment, decision making, orientation to physical surroundings, and language. A working diagnosis of Alzheimer disease is usually made on the basis of the neurological examination. A definitive diagnosis can be made only at autopsy. On a cellular level, Alzheimer's disease is characterized by unusual helical protein filaments in nerve cells (neurons) of the brain. These odd twisted filaments are called neurofibrillary tangles. On a functional level, there is degeneration of the cortical regions, especially the frontal and temporal lobes, of the brain.

Alzheimer's disease is the most common of all neurodegenerative diseases. It accounts for about two-thirds of cases of dementia with vascular causes and other neurodegenerative diseases making up most of the rest.

The average time of survival from the initial diagnosis of Alzheimer's disease was found (in a study reported in 2004) to be 4.2 years for men and 5.7 years for women. Men had poorer survival across all age groups compared with women and survival was decreased in all age groups compared with the life expectancy of the US population.

The German psychiatrist and pathologist Alois Alzheimer (1864-1915) first described this form of presenile dementia in 1907. (German psychiatrist Emil Kraepelin named the disease in his honor.)

Their doctor's recommendation to me at this time was to consider putting them in an assisted living home, because he felt Mom would become more difficult to manage in a home environment, even with Home Health Care. His prognosis for Mom was a survival of 1 ½ years. He felt Dad was at the beginning of the disease. He also recommended putting them on the new drugs at the time for the treatment of Alzheimer's disease, which supposedly slows the progression down. The drugs do not cure it, but in some individuals it slows the progression of the disease.

Faced with the reality of their condition, I knew that I needed to always be planning ahead for them. No longer could I just live day to day in hopes that all this would just suddenly disappear and my parents would no longer need me to take care of them. I knew my journey had just begun. I was scared and turned to God for help.

The next day I was blessed when the Home Health Agency sent me Monica. When she came through the front door of my parents house I was overwhelmed with a feeling that my Grandmother had just walked into the room. Monica's statue, her laughter, her shining light was identical to my grandmother who had passed many, many years ago. Little did I realize that this wonderful woman would soon become my "go to" Mom. She would be the angel sent to me from God when I needed one.

Monica came in and "took-over". She made me laugh when I was crying and as she told me many, many times "you have nothing to cry about, because you have done the best you could do." With Monica now in the house and taking care of Mom and Dad I knew that I could walk away and everything was going to be okay.

July, 2006

Everything finally started falling into place. Monica was my guardian angel for Mom and Dad. I could be home and focus on the many things I still had yet to do. My plans were to return to Mom and Dad's house toward the end of August to celebrate their 61st Wedding Anniversary. With this in mind I had approximately a month and a half to get ready for it.

I wanted it to be a special celebration for them, because I felt this could possibly be the last time they celebrated their 61 years of marriage together. I enthusiastically worked on putting together a collage of photographs of them when they were first married and arranged their marriage certificate along side and framed it to present to them from their family.

I also took advantage of this time to work daily on a scrap book to present to Dad in honor of his services in World War II. I had never done a scrap book and at first was hesitant on doing one, out of fear, of not knowing how to. But, I soon convinced myself that it was for a worthy cause –Dad, my Rock!

Wow, it has been only 5 months in the process of taking care of Mom and Dad and I already felt like an expert at what I was doing. I had mastered reconciling their bank statements, paying their bills and still managed to find time for all their other extra curricular activities, let alone my own personal life.

I was blessed to have a wonderful husband's support throughout this journey. John gave me his broad shoulders to lean on. He held my head up when it was down. He carried me when I needed carrying. He kept our household going when I was not there and he took care of my precious doggies Peanut and Holly during my time away from home. And, I know he gave them lots of hugs and kisses for me. He will always be my knight in shining armor. "Thank you, John, I love you."

August, 2006

What a fun month this was going to be! Not only was it my birthday and John always had such wonderful surprises planned for me, I was soon going to see Mom and Dad and our family would be gathering for their 61st Anniversary celebration.

It felt so good to walk through their front door. The now usual surprised look from Mom of what are you doing here. The hugs and kisses from both Mom and Dad. And, now the hugs and kisses from Monica and the joy that filled the whole house brought me peace. The next several days were a breeze preparing the finishing touches for their party.

My daughter, Courtney arrived shortly after my arrival to help me with everything. Courtney had been driving from Houston to San Antonio every weekend that I was there, giving up her personal time to help me with caring for her Grandfather and Grandmother. She was instrumental in finding all of Mom's loss jewelry that the robbers had supposedly stolen. We spent countless hours analyzing, laughing and crying over many situations that would occur with Mom and Dad. I'm so proud of her and couldn't have gotten through a lot of this without her hugs and beautiful smile. She is a true earth angel and I'm so grateful that she got to participate in a very important part of her grandparent's life with me.

Prior to their party I had arranged for Dad to be examined by a Cardiologist. I mainly wanted Dad to be checked to determine why he was continuing with these dizzy spells. They seemed to be more frequent, or I wondered if he just told me about them, because I was there more often. He was a real trooper when it came time to do all the testing that the cardiologist had him do. We literally spent the entire day there, while he went through every possible test imaginable. When it was all said and done, the doctor came out and told me that Dad had a heart of a 60 year old. There was no blockage and the only thing he could attribute the dizzy spells to was possibly rising too fast from a sitting position. So therefore we instructed Dad to try to rise a little bit slower when he had been sitting for a long time.

This was wonderful news for everyone, and we all felt that Dad would live another 10 years.

The day of their 61'st Wedding Anniversary Party was a busy day. Monica was a jewel with helping me by taking both Mom and Dad for their haircuts. Sue came over early and helped get Mom ready. Mom could no longer dress herself, let alone put on her makeup properly. Sue took pride in her finishing touches on Mom. Mom looked so beautiful. When Dad saw her he did his "wolf" whistle at her like he always would do. She would smile and then scrunch up her face like she didn't believe she looked that pretty. She always had a hard time taking a compliment.

The party began at 4 p.m. and all of Mom and Dad's friends arrived. It was a wonderful party and Mom and Dad thoroughly enjoyed themselves. We took so many wonderful pictures and the memories will be cherished a lifetime, as well as the poem that Dad wrote and sang to Mom that day:

My Loving Wife,

If ever I would leave you……..it wouldn't be in spring time,

Knowing you in spring time I never could go,

No, no, not in spring time, summer, winter or fall,

No never could I leave you at all.

September & October, 2006

It was wonderful to be back home in Virginia. I was able to relax knowing that Monica was taking care of Mom and Dad. They really seemed to enjoy her and she fit in beautiful with our family. When Monica wasn't available to take care of them another wonderful lady name Connie was there. Connie was terrific; she took care of Mom and Dad as if they were her own parents. I was so blessed to have such wonderful people watching over them.

I was able to get a lot accomplished once home and worry free. I had made the decision in August, before I left San Antonio that I would return in November and put on the best Thanksgiving Dinner Mom and Dad had had in a long time. I knew that it had been many years since they had attempted cooking Thanksgiving dinner and once again I had the feeling that this could be their last one together.

I spent these months planning ahead. Planning for any possible future needs for Mom and Dad – not knowing what those would be, but yet accepting that there would be something. I had a very good handle on their finances and with that I knew that I needed professional help with stretching their monies as far as possible. John arranged for us to meet with an Elder Law Attorney. She prepared for us a 5 year plan on how long their money would last by following her guidelines. By far the most cost affective scenario was to keep them in their home which was already paid for and continue with a Home Health Agency, as we had already in place. This plan would work the best, as long as their physical and mental health allowed.

The second plan was to put them in an Assisted Living Facility and run their money down which at that time they would qualify for Medicaid. Medicaid allows an individual to have no more than $2000.00 before they will start paying for any care. This care then needs to take place in a Medicaid Certified Nursing Home. Medicaid will not pay for care in an Assisted Living Facility. All Assisted Living Facilities are private pay. No matter what direction I decided to take, their Estate would need to be evaluated every year to determine if the direction we were moving in was the best for them with whatever money they had remaining.

When I was in Texas in April and August I had visited several Assisted Living Facilities. In April, Dad and I had talked about them moving out of the house. He felt it was just too much for him to take care of. He had been the one doing it for so long. Although, Mom would claim that she was the one still cleaning and cooking, we all knew better. I made arrangements to drive Mom and Dad to a beautiful facility in San Antonio and tour it. They both felt when they walked in to it that all the people were so old in there and that they really didn't belong there. We looked at several models and Mom spent the whole time complaining that the models were too small and there was not enough room to put her entertainment center. I realized how disoriented both of them had become. They were no longer recognizing anything in the neighborhood on our drive. I also felt my father's strong dependence on me at that time. He didn't say anything, but I felt it.

I had also managed in the month of August to visit 2 other facilities. Both of them were more geared to the care of residence with Alzheimer. The facilities were beautiful, and I knew that my parents would eventually adjust. It was depressing though to walk through the Alzheimer care units and see the residence in their different stages of the disease and I knew that someday this too would be my parents.

Being back home in Virginia I also visited several facilities. I had the feeling afterwards that if you've seen one, you've seen them all. I would later learn that this is not true. I realized that through my searching here in Virginia that I was leaning in the direction of bringing my parents to live here. I felt that this would be the best thing for them and it was also one of Dad's requests. He wanted to move back home – home being the northeast. Mom and Dad were born in Pittsburg, PA and like I told him, the next best thing I could do for him was move in to Virginia. "Virginia is for Lovers" and him and Mom were such lovers. They would spend what seemed like ten minutes just staring at one another, each blowing a kiss to the other. It warmed my heart to see this, and I realized then that they were just as much in love with one another today as the day they first met.

On September 1, 1946 they were married in Erie, Pa. Their courtship was pretty much kept a secret from my mother's father, because she was forbidden to date. He insisted that after school she come straight to his tailor shop and work. My grandmother was aware of their dating and even packed them a big picnic basket for them to take with them after they were married, because they left Pittsburg, PA and drove to Corpus Christi, Texas to make this their home. My father told me that he had only $30 and the picnic basket and the reason they chose Corpus Christi, Texas was because he had an army buddy there. They had to run from my mother's father. I found a letter that my father had written to his parents regarding this.

Dearest Mom & Pop

Once again I'm writing to you – seems like old times.

You now should know that Betty and I have run off to get married! I'm sorry Mom and I have to run away like this – I don't like to but there is absolutely no other way – he didn't want us to be together at all – he made us sneak around like a thief so Betty and I could see one another. Mom we couldn't go on like that. Betty and I wanted to be together, to go out twice a week like other young couples do, but he wouldn't let us – so there was nothing else to do but to run away and be married – instead of doing it the right way like Betty and I wanted it. We have planned this for about three months now – and tried our best to keep it secret. I hope he doesn't find out about it until we are married some time today (Sunday). I can't say where we are going because we know he would come after us – so Mom if you don't hear from me for a few weeks – don't be worried.

I'm sorry Mom – but you see now why I wasn't in to big a hurry to get a job – I'm sorry I can't stay here and work for Bell Telephone. I know I would have liked it very much. If there was some other way Mom, we wouldn't run away – but we have thought of every way – please don't be to mad at me and wish us a little luck – cause I know we will need it.

I love you Mom & Pop, Eddie

P.S. Don't let him say bad things about Betty and I – I know that he will, but we didn't do one single thing to be ashamed of.

Bye, Bye, Eddie

Sixty one years later, three children, 3 grandchildren and six great grandchildren they are still as much in love as they were on September 1, 1946 when they married and started their journey of life together. God had a plan for them and it was to travel to Corpus Christi (translation "Body of Christ") and begin a family. My grandfather eventually got over his anger toward them, especially when my Mom started having us babies. We were just too irresistible to our grandfather and next thing we knew my grandmother and grandfather moved to Corpus Christi to be close to all of us. This was God's way of blessing all of us.

November, 2006

I traveled back to Texas and was greeted with lots of hugs and kisses. This time, I had to walk over to Mom who was sitting in her chair. She appeared happy to see me, but seemed to have a difficult time expressing herself. It was then that I noticed how rapidly she seemed to be declining in the disease process. Dad seemed to be the same. There was no drastic change with him. He was still experiencing his dizzy spells and spent most of his day in his T.V. room. What made him happy, made me happy.

It was great catching up with Monica. She was wonderful at reporting to me their every move. She had started expressing to me months earlier that they needed to move out of their house. Mom's dependence on everyone was even more so and there were safety concerns. I knew this would be the time that the decision would be made to either move into an Assisted Living Home or move to Virginia.

John arrived several days before Thanksgiving to help me prepare everything. Courtney had also arrived early to spend time with me. It was great having them there and no doubt their help was needed and appreciated. One afternoon we were all sitting out on the patio and Mom had asked John to get her a coke. John got up, walked into the kitchen, open the refrigerator door, pulled out a coke and walked back out onto the patio. He accomplished this in about 5 seconds. Just as soon as he stepped out on the patio Mom looked up at him and said "What Are You Doing Here". He handed her the coke and we all broke out laughing.

Thanksgiving Day was a wonderful time. It was on this day that I realized the importance of living one day at a time. I could no longer worry about what tomorrow would bring and definitely not worry about what could have been. The most important part of this day was being right here with my family and enjoying every second of this day.

It was decided then that Mom and Dad would move to Virginia. Dad was very excited about it and Mom tried her best to be a part of this conversation. It is sad to see how the disease robs your memory. It truly is a living death. Yet, on this day I was not going to allow the disease to rob me of my joy. I was so grateful and felt so blessed that my parents were still here with me and so thankful to God for blessing me with a wonderful family.

December, 2006

Prior to leaving Mom and Dad's house, Courtney and I spent one day decorating it for Christmas. We put out all of their decorations that they had stored in the closet and probably had not had out in years. It was fun and Mom sat in her chair observing all the activity. I could feel her mind working overtime wanting to tell me where to put what. Wow, I was finally able to do something without my Mom telling me how to do it. Dad even had a twinkle in his eye like a little kid at Christmas when he came into the living room and it was all decorated. I knew on this day of decorating, that this would be their last Christmas together.

I spent the month of December shopping and decorating my two houses. It was a wonderful distraction and "yes" I do love Christmas. What I love about Christmas the most is the decorations, the food and time spent with family. That is the true meaning of Christmas, just as my father had preached to me all those years of growing up. Not giving presents, not receiving presents, but the time you spend with family.

With the houses looking so beautiful and feeling so warm, I allowed myself to enjoy this holiday and set aside my nagging and persistent way I am with myself on needing to get organized for the arrival of Mom and Dad. I was constantly reminding myself to stay in the present.

We decided that we would move Mom and Dad to Virginia in the month of March. This would allow me plenty of time to prepare for it.

I knew it was going to be a lot of work, a lot of hard work, but yet I felt the hardest part of all of this was being away from Mom and Dad until then.

January, 2007

I knew that I had several months to prepare for moving my parents from Texas to Virginia. It was if I went into auto pilot and each day was spent to its fullest. If I stopped long enough to think about this major undertaking of transporting two individuals with Alzheimer disease, as well as my father with his dizzy spells, I would have said I was crazy. I knew that I was on a mission from God. Sounds silly, but I was.

First things first, find them a place to live that would be safe given their condition and that would be close to my home. I would have brought Mom and Dad here to my home, but there were too many safety issues. I live in a 3 story home and there would be no way that they could maneuver the stairs. Mom was already to the point that she needed assistance with all of her daily living activities and Dad was so unstable on his feet.

I had decided to move them into a one story apartment that was equipped to handle them physically. I had found a beautiful place within a mile from my home. This place was safe, being that they were going to be on a first floor only and it was an apartment inside a building, so access outside led into a hallway, which added additional security.

After securing the place I then went and purchased new furniture for them. The decision was made that it would be cheaper to purchase new furniture then to move their furniture that they had in Texas. My plan was to only bring their personal belongings and select trinkets that they would be able to recognize.

I had also interviewed several Home Health Agencies in the immediate area and secured one that I felt would best fit their needs. My father also was a big influence on my decision to go with an apartment instead of an Assisted Living Facility. He was very strong headed about holding on to his independence. As a dutiful daughter, I did my best to oblige him. Mom would come in and out of understanding what was about to happen to her. At the time I felt the biggest adjustment would be on her. I had also felt that Dad would adjust wonderfully to his new surroundings based on his excitement of wanting to move.

February, 2007

Monica called me weekly to keep me up to date with what was happening back in Texas with Mom and Dad. She was instrumental in getting the house ready for the movers. The move date was set for March 28th.

The month of February was spent preparing for two moves. I arranged change of address forms, notified utility companies of shut-off dates in Texas and turn-on dates in Virginia. I closed bank accounts in Texas and opened bank accounts in Virginia. I had medical records from Texas transferred to Virginia. I arranged for doctor appointments with new doctors here in Virginia.

I had arranged also to take possession of their new apartment this month. This would give me time to have the new furniture delivered and setup, as well as do some decorating. The place was finally taking shape and I knew that they would love it when they walked in the door.

I secured airline tickets for myself, Mom, Dad and their Chihuahua, Poncho. The airline required that Poncho be completely up to date on his shots and I had to bring all necessary papers showing this. Because he is small he was allowed to travel inside the plane with us, which means buying a crate that meets airline regulations of being able to fit under the seat. I also alerted the airline that I would need wheelchair assistance in San Antonio, Houston and Virginia. We would be changing planes in Houston and I knew there would be no way that I could push two people in a wheel chair, let alone carry a dog in a crate.

My plan was to head back to Texas the second week of March, which I knew would allow time to coordinate the move at that end. John would be here in Virginia to take care of anything that may arise at their apartment, plus he was going to be the one meeting the movers from Texas when the rest of their belongings arrived.

March, 2007

March had finally arrived and I was so excited and so was Dad. We had spoken weekly on the phone since he had last seen me in November of last year. He was always so positive when I talked with him. He was looking forward to his new home. When I arrived at their home in Texas I got extra hugs and kisses. I observed the progression of the disease was moving a lot quicker in my Mom. My Dad appeared the same, just complained a little bit about dizziness and more unsteadiness on his feet.

I spent the first several weeks going through their remaining belongings. I knew that only so much could come to their new place, because they were going from a 3 bedroom home to a 2 bedroom apartment that was half the size of their home. All important items were ready to be boxed and moved. What the family didn't want, we sold. What we did sell offset the cost of their move.

My main objective was to make it as smooth of a transition as possible for them. I knew that the move would be difficult on them and it was important that their new place have enough familiar stuff in it as possible. I had used the guidance of The Alzheimer's Association to guide me through moving someone with Alzheimer's.

Mom seemed to be handling it fine. She would become curious every so often and would start looking in boxes. We would just simply guide her away from it and tell her to leave things alone and just sit and watch. She took direction from us very well. Dad pretty much stayed in his T.V. room until the movers came and took his T.V. He then had to move out to the living room where we kept the T.V. there. As I had mentioned a lot of the items were remaining behind.

On March 27th the movers arrived. It took them approximately 3 hours to move everything onto the truck. I had purchased new bedroom and living room furniture for my parents. Their old stuff was staying behind and was sold to Mom and Dad's caregivers. I was very blessed that the evening before we were to fly to Virginia that everyone got to sit in the living room and watch T.V. and then retire to their bedroom for a good night sleep.

The next morning I was awake at 4:30 a.m. Monica arrived at 6:00 a.m. to help me get Mom ready for her travel day. We had a nice breakfast and Monica kept us all laughing as she always managed to do. The taxi was scheduled to pick us up at 8:00 a.m. for our 10:30 a.m. departure.

I could tell that Dad was nervous, although he would never admit it. He did a lot more fidgeting then normal and asked me a thousand questions about whether I had secured the house properly and given their neighbor a key, etc., etc.

I learned a long time ago the importance of keeping notes. I kept a pad and pen with me at all times. When caring for someone with Alzheimer it become very distracting and believe me there were many times that I thought I was catching the disease. If I had not written things down the minute I thought of them, I would have forgotten them.

The cab arrived and it seemed to take forever to get Mom and Dad in the cab. Monica was crying, I was crying and Dad even shed some tears. Dad knew as he was getting into the cab he would never see Monica again. Mom was saying her goodbyes too, but I know that there was no way she comprehended what was going on. She was a trooper though and just sat there and kept a sweet smile on her beautiful face. Their dog, Poncho was the only one that seemed excited. I was sad for them, knowing that they would never see their home again. I was scared for them, not knowing what the future held. I was blessed though, having my Mom and Dad right beside me and bringing them home to Virginia to be close to me.

When we arrived at the airport it took awhile before the airline managed to get organized on two wheelchairs. With Mom and Dad finally seated I proceeded to check us in, which appeared to take forever. When we got to the security line, they pushed the wheelchairs around the metal detector and carted my parents off to an enclosed area where they started practically strip searching them. I had to go through the metal detector with the dog and by the time I reached this area I could see my parents confused and struggling with trying to get their shoes off. I was furious to say the least and explained to the security agents that my parents had Alzheimer and did not take direction very well and I needed to help them. They would not let me in this little area. I pitched a huge fit and finally an agent with a kind heart took notice and helped my parents, and this was even after I said my father was a World War II veteran. The Transportation Security Agency that work at our nations airports need to revamp their agency. I have done my share of traveling and over and over again I see them pulling aside the elderly and going through their luggage and practically strip searching them.

There are far more suspicious looking characters out there than the elderly and never once have I seen any of them pulled to the side and put through what my parents had to go through.

Our plane ride from San Antonio to Houston was only 30 minutes and when we arrived in Houston they had wheelchairs waiting for us to take us to our next plane. For the most part Mom and Dad seemed to be handling everything fine. Mom would ask over and over where we were going. She was mostly concerned about holding her dog on her lap. Dad seemed to be getting tired and on several occasions I tried to get him to nap on the plane. The plane landed in Virginia at 5:00 p.m. John was there to greet us and had prepared a wonderful dinner for us at the house.

Mom and Dad's first night in Virginia would be spent at our house. I had figured that it would be good for them to get a good night sleep before taking them over to see their new home.

The first night we all retired early. I was exhausted from traveling all day with Mom and Dad. Everyone seemed to settle down for the night until I awoke to a pounding sound which was coming from the bedroom they were sleeping in. As I approached the door to open it, I noticed that Dad was sleeping on the sleeper sofa in the bedroom next door. As tall as he was he looked a pitiful site with his legs hanging over the edge. I opened the door to the bedroom where the pounding sound was coming from and there laid Mom on the floor pounding on the wall. She was totally disoriented and was wondering where Dad had gone to. God love her, she had no idea where she was. This all occurred at 2:00 a.m. which needless to say I never went back to sleep. Mom wanted to stay awake at this point and I knew that Dad desperately needed his sleep. So did I, but I'm younger and knew I would survive.

Dad came downstairs around 7:00 a.m., looking a little more refreshed. He appeared to be anxious to go see their new home. I was anxious to show it to him. I knew Mom really had no comprehension of where she was going or why. After breakfast, with John's help we got Mom and Dad in the car and drove to their new home. Dad was very impressed and Mom was "just there". I had planned that day to stay with them the whole day and even spend the night. I felt that it would be the best thing because Mom needed constant watching at this point and prior to them arriving in Virginia I had arranged for a home health agency to come in to take care of them. They were not going to start until the next day.

The day in their new home seem to be going fairly well. Mom would ask repeated questions of where was her car. This question was repeated over and over. She could not grasp the fact that we sold it back in San Antonio. God love her and God give me the strength to stay patient. There are many, many times while caretaking I would find myself becoming very impatient. From everything that I read on the subject of caretaking this was to be expected. That is why it is so important to walk away and take time for you.

I spent the day trying to keep them on the same routine they had at their home in Texas. Most of the day was spent watching TV and just visiting. It was wonderful to finally have them here with me. I felt a sense of security that everything would be okay now. I prepared one of their favorite dinners of roasted chicken, mashed potatoes and peas. John was there with us and we all retired to the couch to watch their favorite program "Wheel of Fortune". Afterwards, we had a huge piece of chocolate cake and ice cream and John left to go home, as I stayed to watch them until the next morning when the home health agency would arrive to take over.

That evening around 7 pm I prepared Mom for bed. This was a major undertaking because she could no longer take off her clothes or put on her pajamas by herself. She had reached the stage of Alzheimer's where she needed assistance with all physical activities. After I got her in bed and gave her hugs and kisses she seemed to be so tired I hoped she would stay down the rest of the night. I was exhausted too, but returned to the living room to watch TV with Dad and visit. Dad was happy to be here in Virginia. He was very appreciative of everything John and

I had done to get them here. With the kind words he spoke to me that evening I had a peaceful reassurance that I did the right thing. Once again, that sense of security returned inside of me. Little did I realize at the time that it would be short lived. The truth about caretaking anyone with Alzheimer was to constantly be alert to anything and everything and expect change for the worse.

Dad and I retired to bed at 8 pm. I was exhausted and fell asleep quickly. I left my bedroom door open so I could stay alert to any strange noises. Mom and Dad's bedroom door was closed. That night before going to bed I secured all locks on the front and back door. At 2:00 am I awoke to use the restroom. When I passed their bedroom the door was still closed and upon returning to my bedroom I glanced over at the front door. Dear God the front door was unlocked. I walked over to it and locked it and then returned to my bedroom. As I lay in bed still very sleepy I pondered why the front door was unlocked. I was convinced I locked it, but then wondered if sometime during the middle of the night Dad got up to use the bathroom and confused the front door with the bathroom door. A million thoughts entered my mind as to why the front door was unlocked. It was as I was in shock and my body could not get out of bed. I finally came to my senses and got out of bed and opened their bedroom door only to discover my worst nightmare of Mom not being in the bed. Dad was lying very peacefully and fully asleep, but where was Mom. I immediately fell to my knees and looked under the bed. No Mom. I opened the closet door and looked all around in it, but no Mom. I then quietly closed the bedroom door and ran out the front door into the hallway of the apartment complex, still no Mom. I had selected this particular apartment complex for the reason that all apartment front doors led into an enclosed hall way. The doors leading outside were very hard to open. It required pushing on a bar in order to open. My mother did not have the strength, let alone she could barely walk. Oh my god where did she go? I ran up and down the corridor and still no Mom. There were a total of 6 apartments leading out into this corridor and Mom and Dad were the first residence with only two other apartments being occupied. I went to every door and checked to see if it would open. None did. I then went back inside Mom and Dad's apartment and called John first and then 911. All of this was accomplished in approximately 3 minutes.

John arrived at the same time the police arrived, which was less than 5 minutes. I was by then totally insane with fear of where Mom was. My worst fear of her being outside. Our temperature that evening was in the low 40's. She was only wearing a light weight nightgown. Dear God she would freeze to death. My second worse fear hit me when I visualized in my mind that on one side of this apartment complex was a stream, not to mention the huge swimming pool out back of their apartment. It was after John and the first police officer arrived that I went into their bedroom to wake Dad. Needless to say he was devastated and I watched 20 years come off his life when I told him that Mom was missing. John immediately started searching the apartment grounds which consisted of over 900 apartments. Approximately 20 police officers were doing the same inside and out. One particular officer in charge that night stayed with me asking me all kinds of questions. When did I last see her? What was she wearing, what color was her hair, how tall, any distinguishable scars on her? The officers and John went door to door banging on each one of them. But, how is a deaf person going to hear their banging. Yes, Mom is deaf when she does not have her hearing aides on. The Loudoun County police department then called in reinforcements from Fairfax County. Fairfax County brought in their infra-red helicopter to search the surrounding grounds. They brought in their blood hound dog and just as I went to get the pillow case off of the pillow Mom was sleeping on a police officer came through the door stating that they found her.

This did not occur for 4 hours later when Mom came walking out of the model home apartment carrying an armful of pillows. With tears running down both Dad and my eyes we were so happy to see her and know she was safe. Apparently she had made her way down the hall and found this particular door unlocked and walked in and made herself at home. The funny part of all of this is that she locked the door behind her and when she saw all of us come running up to her she said "well look at everyone who has come to see me". She had the biggest smile on her face and even though she could not hear, she acted as if she could.

Needless to say I never went back to sleep. Dad did, but Mom stayed awake for me to watch until home health arrived that morning at 11 am. Thank the lord that they were there to relieve me, because I knew I needed to step away. I was tired and my patience was just about gone. Mom and Dad seemed to like the caretaker that had arrived to take over. I don't even remember the drive home to my house. I tried my best to lay down on my bed and rest, but I couldn't. It was deep rooted in me now that staying on guard at all times was a fact of life for me now.

I returned back to their apartment that afternoon around 5 pm to relieve their caretaker for the evening. This would continue for approximately 2 weeks until they were able to find a caretaker who would stay with Mom and Dad full time. It was a fact of life, a necessary fact of life. The safety issues that arise with someone with Alzheimer were just being learned by me. I knew from this day forward Mom could never be left out of anyone's sight. And I knew from this day forward that Dad would never leaver her out of his sight.

April, 2007

Finally, with a full-time caretaker in place I thought I could relax, let my guard down a little bit. I tried my best to bring some joy to the situation that what appeared to be some sense of fear in Dad. I took him on outings as much as he would allow to be separated from Mom. I spent everyday at their apartment and everyday that I left to come home my Dad would ask me how soon I would be back. I knew he was dependent on me for his own security. This made it harder and harder for me to stay away, because all I wanted was his peace of mind. As the weeks went by Dad started complaining about everything. He never was one to complain and was always so laid back. As he would always say to me "don't make a big deal about it Debbie", but yet here he was making a big deal about everything. He didn't like the caretaker, complained about her, her cooking, her accent and not being able to understand her. He worried over the alarm system that we installed on both doors. His adjustment was not going very well for him and I kept telling myself that it would take some more time.

We had only kept the first caregiver for 2 weeks and then the second one started. She appeared fine to me, but my Dad had an issue with her also. I had come to realize that he was going to have issues with everyone, because it was not me taking care of them. Somehow, I told myself he would just have to get over it and adjust, because I could only do so much and be in one place at one time. I had my own home and family I needed to be with. Dad knew this and would apologize to me constantly about his behavior, but yet he just couldn't seem to get it under control.

This month was also spent getting acquainted with their new doctor here in Virginia. He spent more time with Dad then he did with Mom. It was sad to see him just kind of pass over Mom like she was not even there. It was agreed by both of us at the time that Mom was just to be maintained and kept comfortable. He felt Dad's cognitive skills were still pretty good and we both felt he could live another 10 years. A second doctor's opinion reassured me that Dad had some years left on him. I made another change with a caretaker at the request of Dad. This time I found a lady who was independent and lived in another state. We interviewed her and she seemed excellent for the job. She spoke excellent English and had a good strong voice that I knew could be heard by Dad, as well as Mom. With her in place I finally felt like I could relax a little and take care of myself. Everything that I had read on the subject of Alzheimer stressed over and over the need to take care of you. Our new caretaker only lasted 2 weeks. I was walking into my doctor's office when she called me to tell me that she could no longer do the job. I asked why and she said it was just too stressful. When I got inside my doctor's office I collapsed. It was as if my whole world had fallen apart. What was I going to do? So many tears poured out of me that morning in the doctor's office. I felt embarrassed by my reaction to her quitting, but also realized that it was many, many months of stress building inside of me. I was no expert at what I was doing. I was trying as fast as I could to read as much about caretaking and as much about the subject of Alzheimer as I could. Hoping that any piece of information would make it easier, would somehow make it all go away and that somehow my Mom and Dad would just be normal again and could take care of me in my time of need.

With a slap of reality, I sucked it up and realized that my job was just beginning and most important to me at the time was keeping my parents as comfortable and as safe as I possibly could. I knew that there was peace missing in my Dad and I was determined to find it for him. I knew he was afraid and I knew that he knew he could no longer protect Mom like he once was able to do. That is why he was leaning on me so strongly.

"Dear God, give me the strength, the courage and the compassion needed for this job."

May, 2007

The few days left in March and the first few weeks of April were spent sleeping at their apartment, while the home health agency provided me with a caretaker for the day. It was in the first week of this month that I knew I needed to make a change to move them from this apartment into an assisted living home. This was something Dad seemed to resist for sometime and the main reason they were not in one from the beginning of their move here to Virginia.

One day when Dad and I were out driving I took him over to visit a reputable assisted living facility close to my home. I had researched many facilities here in Virginia and this one appeared to be a good fit for their needs. As Dad and I walked through the halls and visited with the other residents, I could see a reassurance in Dad that Mom would be safe there. It was explained to him that the doors are locked and a person sits at the front desk watching the door all the time. He finally agreed that this was the place to move to, which the move-in date was set for May 11th.

This gave me less than 1 week to hire movers and move them to their new home, which consisted of one large room of living space. All that could be moved into their new home were their clothing and bedroom furniture. I had an entire apartment full of brand new furniture to now sell, not to mention all the kitchenware and personal things that were brought from Texas.

With the help of John we pulled it off. Mom and Dad moved into their Assisted Living Facility without a hitch and John instrumented an estate sale of their remaining furniture. All personal items were brought to our home.

I was once again exhausted, but yet excited for their new beginning and hoped and prayed to God that all would go smooth from this day forward. Dad and especially Mom were adjusting beautifully within the first few days at their new place. They were making friends, enjoying the food and finally adjusting when just three days after moving in – Dad was being rushed to the emergency room.

The call from the facility came here to my home at 1 pm that day and when I saw the number on caller id my heart stopped. I was told that Dad was being transported to the emergency room. That he had falling and his behavior was very erratic and had been most of the morning. When I arrived at the emergency room they had him hooked up to all kinds of monitors and were assessing him. His blood pressure was very high and even climbed to 208/102. He was admitted to the hospital for further testing which later was determined he had a Transient Ischemic Attack (TIA). **What is a TIA or transient ischemic attack?** A TIA is a "warning stroke" or "mini-stroke" that produces stroke-like symptoms, but no lasting damage. Recognizing and treating TIAs can reduce your risk of a major stroke.

Most strokes aren't preceded by TIAs. However, of the people who've had one or more TIAs, more than a third will later have a stroke. In fact, a person who's had one or more TIAs is more likely to have a stroke than someone of the same age and sex who hasn't.

TIAs are important in predicting if a stroke will occur rather than when one will happen. They can occur days, weeks or even months before a major stroke. In about half the cases, the stroke occurs within one year of the TIA. **What causes a transient ischemic attack?** TIAs occur when a blood clot temporarily clogs an artery, and part of the brain doesn't get the blood it needs. The symptoms occur rapidly and last a relatively short time. Most TIAs last less than five minutes. The average is about a minute. Unlike stroke, when a TIA is over, there's no injury to the brain. **What are the symptoms of a TIA?**

It's very important to recognize the warning signs of a TIA or stroke. The usual TIA symptoms are the same as those of stroke, only temporary:

- Sudden numbness or weakness of the face, arm or leg, especially on one side of the body
- Sudden confusion, trouble speaking or understanding
- Sudden trouble seeing in one or both eyes
- Sudden trouble walking, dizziness, loss of balance or coordination
- Sudden, severe headache with no known cause

The short duration of these symptoms and lack of permanent brain injury is the main difference between TIA and stroke.

I arrived home that night around 10:30 pm only to get a phone call to come back to the assisted living home and get my parents dog because he would not allow anyone to get close to my mother. Poncho, their Chihuahua had become very aggressive and protective of her. I wasn't even sure he would let me put a leash on him, but he did and was more then happy to leave the place and get outside to go to the bathroom. I found out later that he stayed in their bedroom all day. Poor thing needed to go potty. I brought Poncho home and knew at this time that it was time to find another home for Poncho. I knew that Mom was incapable of taking care of him and I did not know what condition

Dad would be in and even when he would return to the assisted living facility.

With John's help we contacted Chihuahua Rescue here in Virginia and took him to them. Happy to say they were able to immediately place him. This was the best decision we made at the time. It had become more and more difficult for Dad to walk Poncho. Dad was already very unstable on his feet and constantly suffering from dizzy spells. Now we knew why. The mini strokes were gradually taking its toll on him and as the doctor told me it would be a matter of time before the major one.

Four days after entering the hospital Dad was allowed to leave. They put him on medication to thin his blood, as well as a mild anti-depressant to help him with his mood swings. He was sad when I told him about Poncho, but quickly dismissed it as the right thing to do. He was more concerned about Mom missing Poncho, but she never really mentioned it until one day we were sitting out on the front porch and she put her arms together as if she was holding a baby and said "I use to have a baby". This is how she would hold Poncho, just like she was holding a real baby. I don't know and will never know if she really meant Poncho or meant one of us kids. If I allowed myself to think about it too long I would become sad and my job was to stay positive and keep a smile on my face and just get through one day at a time.

With Mom and Dad together again the remainder of the month was uneventful. "Thank you, God." We spent this month adjusting and meeting new people that lived at the facility. I came to realized how fortunate I was when I saw the later stages of Alzheimer's in some of the other residents. At least I could still make my Mom laugh and I could still understand the words she spoke to me. I prayed for these moments to last as long as they could. I knew from all my research that this time would pass quicker then I wanted it to, because I already saw the rapid change in my mother from the first day in February, 2006 when I walked in the front door of their house in Texas, to this month of May, 2007. I was just grateful to still have both of them in my life and thanked God every second I could for allowing me to be here with them. Every minute I could I was touching, kissing and hugging them both. Because I knew that someday would come and I would never have this opportunity again.

June, 2007

I was really looking forward to this month. John and I were going on a 2 week trip to Italy and I felt Mom and Dad would be okay where they were now. I tried to get Mom and Dad out of the facility for little outings to my house. They seemed to enjoy this and in the beginning my intentions were to bring them to my house as often as I could. Little did I realize the undertaking of doing so.

Mom was pretty much wheel chaired bound at this point. She would attempt to walk, but was very unstable on her feet, as well. The caretakers at the Assisted Living Home were very concerned about her falling, as well as Dad falling. We tried unsuccessfully to get Dad to even use a cane, let alone a walker and the thought of going in a wheel chair – well, he wouldn't have anything to do with it.

Their outings to my house had to be orchestrated. We first had to make sure there was another male here to help John with getting my mother up the stairs. This literally included them carrying her up the stairs. Then we had to bring the wheel chair up the stairs. I noticed on these times that Mom enjoyed her ride up the stairs, but more important I noticed that Dad needed assistance, as well. He wouldn't admit it, but he was so unstable on his feet. I stayed beside him doing what I could, but knew that if he fell he would take me down with him. I had hoped if that happened he would land on me and somehow I would cushion him from the fall.

They really seemed to enjoy themselves when they were here. The weather was perfect for sitting outside. Dad would enjoy himself a couple of beers with John and Mom would busy herself with my one Chihuahua that looks exactly like her Poncho. She would even call her Poncho and think nothing of it when I would turn to her and call her Holly. It was a relaxing time, although I had to watch Mom like a hawk. Once I rounded the corner to see where she went and there she was in the kitchen sitting in her wheel chair taking off her shirt and just sitting there in her bra. One time we had to stop Dad from putting salt into his water glass. Every time that they were here we had to listen to Mom say "when are we going home". I knew then that she meant the assisted living facility, because as soon as she walked through their doors she had the biggest smile on her face. I knew she had adjusted completely. And, just as soon as I knew that I also felt that Dad was struggling. His complaining once again started. It was slow at first, very subtle, but yet the comments began. I dismissed it at first as him being tired.

My oldest daughter once made a comment to me about the difference between her grandmother and grandfather and her three children. She said to me, "at least I know that my children will outgrow their terrible two's." Her grandparents had a disease that they could not outgrow. I knew that Dad was struggling in his mind with what was real and what was not. I tried my best to help him find balance and peace.

July, 2007

Mom and Dad had only been living in Virginia for four months and everything I had read about Alzheimer's, I felt that they should be now fairly settled into their new way of living. Mom seemed to be well adjusted, but yet the struggle was still with Dad. He would go in and out with his mood swings. I could not understand what was going on, but told myself with time he would adjust and I continued to be as patient as possible. I knew that I had taken him from his home and brought him to a new area that was so unfamiliar to him. I prayed everyday and night to God for his help in helping Dad adjust. I asked God to protect him and guide him to peace.

I had spent the first part of this month at my mountain home. I needed the rest and relaxation and my home in the mountains provided me with such. It was also my way of walking away. My sister and so many other friends and family had told me that I needed to walk away and not be so available to Dad. They all felt that Dad was too dependent on me and by walking away he would adjust quicker. But, my god it had only been four months.

This was also the month that Mom and Dad's best friends Jeff and Laurie Lee came to visit. It was so wonderful having them here. I knew that they would be able to assess Mom and Dad and help me with any future plans. During their visit I was able to open up to Laurie

Lee and express my deepest fears. It was during there visit that I had a feeling deep down inside of me that I didn't have much more time with Mom and Dad. My deepest fear was being alone when their time came to die. I was scared and so scared of not doing the right thing or saying the right thing at their time of death. I just wanted to give my fullest to my mother and father in their time of need and I hoped that this would be the case upon their death. Laurie Lee couldn't give me the words, but she knew what I felt. She had been there before with her own mother.

Mom and Dad were excited to see them. When we arrived at the assisted living home, Dad stood up from his chair and announced to all the residence that they were his very dear friends from Louisiana. He was so proud and excited to be able to show them off. Mom even appeared to recognize them. It was a joyous time.

One day we brought Mom and Dad to my house for a visit. It was during this time that Jeff and Laurie Lee could see the tremendous change in both Mom and Dad, but yet especially in Dad. They noticed the decline in his physical strength. His extreme unstableness when he walked. Our visit at my home was wonderful. Dad, Jeff and John had a couple of beers and it was obvious that Dad was enjoying himself. Mom was just stuck in time, but always kept her pleasant smile on her face. She was so cute and all I ever wanted to do with her was give her kisses. Lots of kisses. When it was time to leave and take them back to the assisted living home Dad became very unstable on his feet. It took Jeff holding him, or else he would have fallen. When we got back to their home, once again he almost fell. It was obvious to Jeff and Laurie Lee that although Dad's mind wanted to keep going, his body no longer could.

The remainder of time that Jeff and Laurie Lee were here was spent relaxing and spending time at our mountain home. I needed it and it was so good to have them here.

August, 2007

I was looking forward to this month. It was not only my birthday month, but my sister was coming to visit. I knew that she would be able to see the changes in Mom and especially in Dad that I have been seeing for over a year. I needed validation from her, just like I had just received from Jeff and Laurie Lee. I was also afraid for what Sue was about to see in Mom and Dad. She hadn't seen them since February and I knew that it would be so difficult on her. How could I shelter her from the pain of what she was about to see.

When she first walked into their room at the assisted living home, there was Dad lying on the bed. She saw him for the first time, just as I had seen him for months laying there on the bed so weak. Our father, always so strong, but yet so weak. Sue asked him if he was dying and his reply to her was "no". Dad always had a way of protecting Sue. He was doing it then and I knew it. Time and time again I found him this way and I knew that he was dying, but yet the reality had not completely sunk in.

Sue and I went daily to visit Mom and Dad. We also managed to spend some alone time at my mountain home. It was so much fun getting away with her and doing the things sisters do, just having fun. God, I needed it. I hated to see her go, because once again I felt alone, unprepared in my mind of what I knew was going to happen.

After Sue left I continued with my daily routine of visiting Mom and Dad. There was this urgency deep inside of me that I needed to be with them daily. I didn't know why, I just knew that I needed to be there. Yes, everyone told me to stay away, but yet Dad needed reassurance that everything was going to be okay. I knew that once I saw this in him, then I could relax. One day when I was visiting them, Dad turned to me and said "I was talking with my father last night and he told me that he too had mini strokes". I prayed to God for his help, because I knew at this very moment Dad's time was near.

September, 2007

This was a busy month for all of us. The decision had been made to move Mom and Dad from the assisted living facility they had been in to another one that was better equipped with taking care of them. Mom had become more difficult to manage and I was concerned with the quality of care she was receiving and found a wonderful place that would provide both of them with the quality of care they needed.

It was also around the last week of August while visiting them prior to their move, Dad asked me not to go anywhere. I had first thought he meant for me not to go to my mountain home and I turned to him and reassured him that I would be beside him daily. He then asked me if Sue would be here. At first I thought he meant would she come for another visit and I reminded him that she had just been here. He sternly turned to me and said in his strong voice "no will she be here". It was at this second I knew what he meant. It was this very day I called Hospice to help me. It was at this last week in August the Hospice doctor told me that Dad had given up and that it was a matter of time. I asked the doctor how much time and he told me in his experience he has seen when someone gives up it can be 6 months to a year. My gut told me it would only be a month.

Hospice is derived from the Latin word *hospitium*, ``hospitality," an inn for travelers, especially one kept by a religious order. The hospice movement was started by Dr. Cicely Saunders in England in the 1940s, when St. Christopher's Hospice was opened to provide a quiet place where people could die in peace and dignity. It was staffed by nuns who had a sense of commitment to service.

Hospice care was introduced in the United States in 1974 at Yale in New Haven, Connecticut. Since then, the movement has expanded rapidly, with programs based on several organizational models: all-volunteer, hospital-based, integrated with home health agencies or freestanding community hospices. Though diverse, these programs share a philosophy.

Despite all the advances in diagnosis and treatment, a cure is not always possible. Continued treatment, even if available, may compromise a patient's quality of life. After discussion with the physician and consideration of treatment options and the potential outcomes, it may be appropriate to consider palliative (comfort) care. Some patients and families are frightened by the word hospice, believing that all treatment will be discontinued and the patient is being sent home to die. But many kinds of treatment may be continued to provide comfort and relief of pain.

The hospice philosophy embraces a holistic approach that encompasses physical, emotional and spiritual concerns. The patient and family are seen as the unit of care. Care has to be individualized to meet the patient's and the family's needs, as well as being responsive to differences in lifestyles. The hospice philosophy:

- Affirms life
- Promotes self-determination, as patients and families participate in their plan of care
- Provides education to help patients and families provide appropriate care

- Promotes understanding and accepting that the journey of life eventually leads to death, and encourages people to view this experience as an opportunity for growth
- Emphasizes palliation, which includes physical, psychological and spiritual comfort delivered by a multidisciplinary staff

When medical treatments have been exhausted or the burden of treatment outweighs the benefits, it may be time to consider hospice care. Most people would like to end their lives surrounded by family and friends. By bringing services into the home, hospices help patients and families provide the necessary care. Patients and families are able to retain a greater sense of control at home than in the hospital. Hospices will also provide services in convalescent homes to ensure pain and symptom management and to provide support to families. The hospice experience can foster spiritual and personal growth as the hospice team empowers patients and families to manage difficult situations.

Some hospices are supported by the community with their own fundraising and donations; other programs have a large volunteer component. Hospices may be incorporated with home health agencies or hospitals, or they may receive funds from foundations and grants. Private health insurance and Medicaid are some other forms of reimbursement. In 1982, Medicare began reimbursing certified Medicare hospices, which must adhere to specific guidelines. Part A of Medicare covers most of the costs.

Dad had been looking forward to the move to the new facility. I had prepared him weeks in advanced and when we talked about it he seemed to be looking forward to it. I had spent weeks getting the new place ready for them. I had been going back and forth between the facilities preparing for the big day.

The morning of September 24th I arrived to pick up Mom and Dad and transport them to their new home. When I arrived I found them both in their bedroom, Mom sitting in her wheel chair and Dad still lying in bed fully dressed. He tried to jump up out of bed, just like he would do every time I came over, but this time he had difficulty doing so. He couldn't even seem to place his feet on the floor. When I tried to assist him, in his stubborn way he told me he needed to go to the restroom. He could barely walk and was holding on to the side of the bed and only made it a few steps before he was clinging to Mom's wheel chair. With my help he made it to the restroom, but then was asking me for scissors to cut his clothing so he could go to the bathroom. I immediately called a nurse to help. When they arrived he seemed to settle down. We said our good byes to the staff and started on our short drive to the new facility. In the car Dad's behavior became strange once again. He became extremely agitated and I prayed to God once again to just get us there safely. His behavior was frightening me.

I had earlier alerted the staff of the new facility that we were on our way and that Dad's behavior was not good. They were waiting for us when we arrived. At this point when we got out of the car Dad could barely walk. We put him in a wheel chair and proceeded to show him around. Mom appeared to be enjoying herself and saying her "hellos" to everyone. Dad was confrontational, paranoid, but yet polite.

When we got to their new bedroom, Dad exploded. He refused to enter the bedroom and the nursing staff and I just obliged. One of the things I had read with Alzheimer patients is not to confront them when they are agitated. I stood back and just observed at this point him looking around, but yet being polite. It was after a while that the staff and I decided for me to leave and just let them settle in. It was 10:30 a.m. when I left and the phone call came in at 11:00. Dad had a melt down. He became very violent throwing things and was now endangering not only himself, but all the other residents. His behavior from earlier that morning had completely flipped. He was now Mr. Hyde!

The nurse who called me informed me that he could not stay there and they were afraid he could hurt the other residents. He had not even made it a day in this new place, what was I going to do, where was I going to take him? The nurse suggested that I check him into the hospital for evaluation. That afternoon, he had settled down after they had given him medication and John and I arrived to drive him to the hospital. He didn't resist going, but only asked who would take care of Mom. I reassured him she would be taken care of. When we arrived at the hospital we waited and waited and waited before he was seen. John entertained him by feeding him Peanut M&Ms and a Dr. Pepper. He was in hog's heaven. Dad always had a sweet tooth. He seemed so peaceful sitting there, while I was sitting on pins and needles wondering what was going to happen next.

After many hours of waiting, Dad was admitted that night into the hospital. I knew that he would never leave the hospital. He knew too. One of the last things Dad said to me that night was "Deb, don't you make a big deal about all of this". God gave me the strength that night to be as brave as I could be for him. I kept the tears away from him, or else he would have felt my broken heart. I kept the tears away from him, or else he would have felt my fear of taking care of Mom without him beside me. "Daddy don't leave me, you're my rock that keeps me strong".

John and I left him at 2:00 am in the morning the next day. As exhausted as I was, I didn't sleep. I laid there in bed accepting the future and praying to God to guide me to be the best that I could be for my father as he nears the end of his life. I knew that God had chosen me and with God beside me now I would hold Dad's hand as far as I could.

I spent the next several days going back and forth between Mom and Dad. I had called Sue to prepare her for what I knew was about to happen. She made plans to arrive on Monday, October 1, 2007.

October, 2007

The first few days in the hospital I was told that Dad had experienced several more strokes. One of the strokes required 4-5 nurses to hold him down. He became very physical during these episodes and on this particular one he managed to break one of the nurse's glasses. They had him in a room directly outside the nurses' station where they could monitor him 24/7. There was also a nurse brought in from Hospice to sit vigilantly outside his bedroom door. He continued to make attempts at trying to get out of bed, but his body defied him. Because of these attempts he was a tremendous fall risk.

On the Sunday before Sue's arrival I spent 6 hours with Dad sitting beside him and whispering in his ear all my love for him. I told him that I knew he was dying and that I had accepted that he had given up. It was because of this knowledge I asked him if he was ready to accept Jesus into his life and he told me yes. I remember back in August of 2006 sitting outside on the patio with him having the discussion about life after death and it was at that time that he told me he did not believe in such a thing. I turned to him and said then you must not believe in Jesus. He expressed his doubts to me.

I was so happy on that day of Sunday that he finally accepted Jesus into his life. I wondered as I sat next to him, holding his hand if it was because he was afraid of dying, or was it because he finally accepted that death was right around the corner. Nevertheless, I knew on that day that my father was blessed by our lord and that my father would be going to heaven and that he would be joining his son, my brother Danny. I no longer was afraid and I too accepted my father's dying. It also was comforting knowing that Sue was coming and would help me stay strong when I needed it. I knew it was going to be hard for her to accept what she was about to see in Dad, but I also knew that I had prepared her the best I could about our father dying. I prayed that by doing so would make it a tiny bit easier for her to see him in the condition that he was in.

The afternoon of October 1st I picked Sue up at the airport. We went to the house first and had a short visit over a glass of wine. Sue appeared exhausted from traveling, yet I could see the sadness in her knowing that she was about to see Dad. She was afraid, she was sad, just as I had been days before. We drove that evening to the hospital and when we arrived they had Dad sitting up in a chair and they were attempting to give him medications. Just as we were walking in the door he was hollering at the top of his lungs for them to stop and then he hollered "please respect my dignity, no more pills". It was at that point I knew and so did Sue they needed to stop forcing anything and everything into his mouth and our intention was to speak with the doctor first thing the next day.

I left Sue alone to visit with Dad. It was very difficult for her seeing him this way. It had only been several months since she had last seen him and it was very clear that he was dying. Dad was a tall man of about 6'1" and weighted at his healthiest weight 180 lbs. He now maybe weighted 150 lbs. His rib cage was protruding to the point you would think it was going to rip through his skin. His arms were covered in bruises from his many bumps and falls prior to entering the hospital, as well as I'm sure from the nurses having to hold him down. His eyes remained closed, just as they had been the day he first entered the hospital. At times when he attempted to open his eyes, it was as if he was blind. His eyes were glassy and no movement. God love him, he still did his best at visiting with Sue and I. He still continued to show his strength of a father that we always knew him as. He was still "my rock". Our visit with Dad that evening wasn't very long, maybe an hour. He got tired easily and Sue and I were both exhausted mentally and I know Sue was physically as well.

The next day we got to the hospital in the morning and were fortunate to get to meet with the doctor who we instructed that all medications for Dad were to be stopped. He agreed and it was now determined nothing in the mouth, unless of course Dad accepted it or wanted it. We all tried our best to get Dad to drink a little water, eat a little food, but he slowly refused it all. Each day that we visited we saw him become weaker and frailer. On Saturday, October 6th Sue, John and I visited Dad. It was on this day that John told Dad that he did not need to worry about a thing and that it would be his job now to take care of me, Sue and Mom. I knew that this brought Dad much comfort. He even ate a little bit of chocolate ice cream for John. It was the only thing he had eaten in days. It was decided on Sunday, October 7th that we would say our goodbyes to Dad. Sue would be leaving on Monday. It was a very difficult thing to do, but as I explained to Sue and my daughter Kellye, Dad needed to know that we would be okay after his death. I had read through Hospice that so many dying people hold-on until their family comes forward and says their goodbyes. My daughter Kellye had gone first and we respected her privacy and left the room. She shared with him her "near death" experience she had had. I knew her Pop Pop was listening to her and I also knew how difficult it must have been for the both of them. Her knowing she was saying goodbye to her grandfather and him knowing he was about to leave his first granddaughter.

Sue went next. We respected her privacy and left the room. I knew whatever words she was about to speak to him would be words that would break her heart and just as she too was trying to stay strong through expressing her goodbye's that her father too was being strong for her as he held her hand as long as he could. I knew it really brought no comfort to Sue to have to say goodbye to Dad. I wished that I could have just waved a magic wand on this day and spared everyone the pain. Yet, through it all I knew God was guiding us through this day and helping us with our words.

When it was my turn, I repeated my words to Dad that I had done the past Sunday by telling him I loved him so very much and that I would always remember him and would never forget him. I thanked him for raising me to be the compassionate person I am today, as well as I asked him for his forgiveness in all the miserable times I knew I had put him through as a daughter, but yet I knew he agreed with me when I told him I certainly had made up for those times. I asked him to say hello to Danny for me and to give him a big, strong hug from me and to also tell him that someday, I too would be with him. I kissed Dad on his cheek and told him it was okay to go and that he would finally be at peace.

Monday morning, October 8th Sue and I went to visit Mom before I was to take her to the airport. Her flight was to leave at 1 p.m. this day and we figured to spend a couple of hours with Mom before she had to go. Our visit was good. Mom appeared upbeat and seemed to recognize Sue. We had a good visit and Sue said her goodbyes to Mom. I knew it would be her last time to see our Mom. I think Sue knew it too.

After I dropped Sue off at the airport I stopped by Kelley's work and picked her up to go grab a bite to eat and then go to the hospital to see Dad. Even though we said our goodbyes yesterday, it was extremely difficult for me to stay away. I just wanted to see him and most important know that he was not suffering.

When we were about to walk into his room the nurses were turning him on his side. He became very agitated by this, just as he had done many times before and in a clear and demanding voice asked them to stop. After they left the room, Kellye and I walked in. Kellye stood at the foot of his bed and I went to his side. When I reached for his hand, he flung it, almost as if telling me to leave. He was already lying on his back and his head was slightly turned toward the wall and he had his eyes open, fixed and staring up towards the ceiling as if he was having a very intense conversation with someone. I held his hand for a brief moment, kissed him on his cheek and told him I loved him. I had an overwhelming feeling that I was invading his privacy. It was after my kiss to his cheek that I turned away and cried out to God to please not let him suffer and Dear God I could not return the next day, by myself and see him the way he was, pure skin and bones. As I drove Kellye home she told me that she too had the feeling that Dad did not want us in the room.

After I dropped her off, I cried all the way home. I asked God to please not let Dad suffer anymore and please bring him home. I spoke to God my fears of being by myself through the process of death and having to return to the hospital another day. My fear of being alone had return.

That evening I shared my feelings with John and I also thanked God for having such a wonderful man by my side. As I lay beside him that night I prepared myself for the phone call that I knew would come. It had not even made it to the second ring when John answered it. I knew from that first ring what I was about to hear on the other end of the line. I knew that the call was to tell me that Dad had passed. I spoke with the nurse who told me she was beside Dad when he passed. She was a very compassionate person and even thanked me for allowing her to be beside him at his time of death. She told me that Dad went very peacefully, taking one last breath. She told me that she worked the night shift and she would sit beside Dad every night and comfort him. She was an angel sent to him in his final hours. Several days before Dad's passing I had already contacted the Funeral home where Dad's body was to be transported to. I had given this information to the hospital. When the hospital called that night John and I had not noticed the time. It wasn't until we were sitting downstairs talking, crying and yes, even feeling relief that it was over for Dad and he was now with our lord that John turned to me and asked me to check our "caller ID" to see what time the call came in. To my astonishment it was at exactly 3:33 a.m. Many months prior to Dad's passing I kept waking at night and upon immediately opening my eyes the first thing that I would see is our clock and it would say 3:33 a.m. I remember after waking and seeing this time over and over that I finally spoke about it to John. I questioned why I was waking to exactly 3:33. One day John called me and told me to go buy a book called "Angel Numbers", written by Doreen Virtue, Ph.D. In her book she explains why we always see the same numbers everywhere we go. In her book she explains that the angels give us messages in the form of number sequences. For example, you may have noticed that you frequently see the same numbers (such as 111, 333 or 444) every time you look at a clock, glance at license plates, or dial phone numbers. I bought her book and was fascinated by what my angels were telling me about the number 333.

333 – You've merged with the ascended masters, and they're working with you day and night – on many levels. They love, guide, and protect you in all ways.

As Doreen explains in her book the number 3 refers to ascended masters, great spiritual teachers who once walked upon the earth. She goes on to explain that when she gives an angel number reading for someone who sees the numeral 3 frequently, she usually finds that Jesus is with that person. Number-sequence interpretation is an easy way to receive messages from your angels. Each number has a unique vibration frequency relating directly to its meaning.

She further explains this ancient wisdom harkens back to great teachers such as Hermes, Plato, and Pythagoras. Pythagoras said that everything in the Universe is mathematically precise, and that each number has its own vibration, meaning, and virtue. Plato wrote that everything in the Universe is built from basic geometrical shapes derived from numbers, such as triangles (from 3) and cubes (from 4). The sacred mystical Jewish text of the Zohar (Kubbalah) discusses the power of the vibrations from numbers and letters.

In her book, Doreen explains the angels also say that the placement of the numbers in a sequence holds special meaning. For example, when there are three or more numbers, the center digit is of primary focus. The angels say that this number represents the "heart" of the matter. Numerology is one of the few sacred sciences that have kept its magic from ancient to modern times. The angels remind us that we're all alchemists, powerful enough to manifest our true desires through Divine magic. Numbers point out the importance of seeing Heavenly messages third-dimensionally in order to show us the lessons, growth opportunities, and guidance contained within each experience.

Just as the book had said "the center digit" which was a 3 represents the "heart" of the matter. When I later looked up the number 3 it said "The ascended masters (such as Jesus) are near. They've responded to your prayers and want to help you.

All along Jesus was beside me guiding me through this experience and answering my prayers for Dad. "Thank you Jesus, but I still need your help, don't leave me now."

I remember the first time my Dad ever mentioned anything to me about when he died what to do with his body. He would jokingly say "just bury me in the compost pit". Our house where I grew up in as a child, he had made a compost pit. Dad always was in his yard working in his garden. Our yard was his pride and joy. And I must admit, even though I didn't pay that much attention to it, I now as an adult can look back and remember how beautiful it was. There were flowers and many tropical plants growing everywhere. He would use the compost for fertilizing his garden. The fruits of his labor no doubt paid off. So it became a standard joke around our house that when Dad died we would bury him in the compost pit.

After Mom and Dad moved from this house he then would say when he dies, just place his ashes in a river. He didn't care what river; just put him in a river. When I moved him and Mom here to Virginia I had decided that the two rivers that flowed through this area were the Shenandoah River and the Potomac River and one of them would serve my Dad's request.

After Dad had passed, the funeral home came and got his body from the hospital and then took it to where it was to be cremated. The next day after Dad had died, John and I went to the funeral home and met with the funeral director to fill out paperwork and discuss services for Dad. While sitting there going over things, I knew the question would come as to what to do with his body regarding burial. I remember feeling awkward and didn't even want to mention that I was going to distribute his ashes into a river. As soon as I did, the funeral director asked me why Dad was not being buried at Arlington Cemetery. I was surprised by his question and told him that I did not think Dad was allowed to be bury there, because he was not an Officer in the Army and I thought only Officers could be buried there. I was told different by the funeral director. He informed me that since Dad's request was to be cremated that he could still be buried in our country's national cemetery. I was overwhelmed with a feeling of how proud Dad would have felt if he knew this. It was at this very moment I knew deep inside that the feeling I was feeling was Dad. So it was decided that this is where he would be laid to rest to be remembered by many generations to come and show their respect to a truly great man. And, the other wonderful part of all of this was that upon Mom's passing, she too would be laid to rest beside him. What an honor. I remember how my father once genuinely thanked someone with "tears" in his eyes when that person turned to him and thanked him for his service to our country. That moment of pride was written all over his face. I knew at this very moment that same "pride" was there, because I could see him smiling and the tears of joy in his eyes.

God once again was right beside me, answering my prayers, holding my hand and showing me that there was nothing to fear. I felt at this time that my going forward with Mom would some how not be as difficult.

Mom's Alzheimer's had progressed so rapidly. Although she could still feed herself, by holding her own utensil from time to time, there were the times she would eat with her fingers, or would become distracted in a split second from the fact that she was just eating. She never lost her socializing skills and would still continue to carry on a conversation with you, even though you didn't understand what she was saying. You just simply nodded your head with a yes, a big smile and even a burst of laughter. Or if it appeared she was talking about something serious, you would just follow her face cues to make your own face in response. There wasn't a day that didn't go buy that I regretted seeing my Mom this way. I enjoyed being with her and knew that each day may be the last. So everyday with her was spent to its fullest. Just sitting beside her holding her hand and not even talking was wonderful. To feel how soft her skin felt, like a new born baby. It is amazing to me how as we age, we return to our beginning of life. God has a plan for all of us. I watched his plan with Dad and now I wanted to watch very, very closely my Mom, not to miss a thing.

Mom knew Dad had passed; she just didn't have the words to express it. Prior to Dad's passing, my sister and I went to visit Mom after we had been visiting Dad. We were sitting there with Mom when all of a sudden she turned to us and said "I'm going to die before you and you and before everyone in this room". It shocked us and what shocked us the most was those were the first clear words she had spoken in months. I remember when she said it I also had a feeling that what she was saying would come true sooner then we wanted it to.

After Dad's passing, Monica came to visit. She was excited to see Mom and when she got there, Mom appeared at times to remember her. Their visit was good and when it came time to leave, as Monica and I were walking out of the nursing home I had an overwhelming feeling that Mom was going to pass within a month. I expressed this to Monica and she felt the same way. It was very comforting to have Monica here for the few days that she was in town. She had provided so much support to me in my times of need. Her smile, her laughter, her words of encouragement gave me strenght.

The remainder of this month I spent everyday visiting Mom. I was fortunate to have her so close to me. I had an unexplained urgency inside of me that everyday was going to be my last with her. Each day that I spent with her I touched her, kissed her in hopes of planting a memory that would last a lifetime.

On Tuesday, October 30th Mom was admitted to the hospital with aspiration pneumonia. The call came into me that night around 11:30 p.m. John and I arrived at the hospital at midnight and found Mom lying on a hospital bed clutching her baby doll. She looked so helpless. "God give me strength."

November, 2007

Mom spent a total of 3 days in the hospital. I made the decision to move her back to the nursing home where she could receive comfort care only by the Hospice team I had been working with. The hospital Mom was in was not setup for Hospice. They were an aggressive treatment hospital, so therefore they were sticking every needle they could in her. She was scared and cried out for her mother many times. I had to fight with the doctor on many occasions as I explained to him Mom was on Hospice comfort care only. This simply means that there would be no aggressive treatment. As long as Mom could take antibiotics by mouth, then fine. But when she continued to pull out her IVs and cried in pain when they re-inserted them I knew I had to put a stop to it and get her out of there. She was dying and I knew it and I would do everything in my power to keep her as comfortable as possible. This hospital was not the place.

When Mom returned to the nursing home she still had pneumonia and was doing a great job at taking her antibiotic. The caretakers would crush the pills and put it into applesauce and she would finish every bit of it. We could definitely see improvement in her mental well being. She was happy to be home and see everyone. She was eating very well the first day back and even ate breakfast her next morning there, but she still was very weak.

On Saturday, day 2 of being back at the nursing home, I went and visited her that morning and stayed until early afternoon. John and I had a dinner party to go to. Mom was very weak and sleeping most of the day. I talked with her and told her that I knew she missed Dad and that she wanted to be with him. I told her that it was okay to go and that I would stay beside her and hold her hand to the very end. At one point I had left the room and walked to the nurses' station to talk with them. They had informed me that she was still eating, but very little. The rule of thumb was as long as she accepted food then give it to her, but no forcing it in her. When I returned to Mom's room she was still lying in bed, just as she had been since she got out of the hospital, but this time she was staring at a picture of my brother on the wall in front of her. Her eyes were fixed on his picture as if she was having a conversation with him. I knew she was and didn't interrupt. She peacefully closed her eyes and appeared to have fallen asleep.

On Sunday morning I was out the door early and there at the nursing home by 9:00. I tried my best to get Mom to eat her breakfast, but she refused, so I didn't force anything. She took several sips of her juice. When the nurse came to give her medicine, she clamped her lips tight and refused her medicine. We knew not to force. Mom continued this behavior from this day on and therefore it was instructed that all medicines would be stopped. On Wednesday she had a little burst of energy. She ate a little scramble egg and drank half glass of orange juice. We tried to dress her, but as soon as we moved her she cried out in pain. She has been in bed for one week and no doubt this was taking its toll on her too. This was when she was given her first dose of morphine. By Friday, they were administering morphine for pain every 6 hours. On Saturday, I said goodbye and gave her permission to die.

By this time Mom had not eaten or drank anything for days and her breathing became more labored, which the nurses then administered an oxygen tank to help ease her breathing. On Tuesday, November 13th when I arrived at 8 a.m. Mom was resting comfortably. That same day my oldest daughter Kellye came to say her goodbye's to her grandmother. Kellye had been there with me toward the end of Dad's life and she was now there with me and Mom. I'm so grateful that God had her there with me. He answered my prayers of not wanting to be alone. I stayed with Mom that day until 9 p.m. I was so afraid to leave, but yet so tired. I knew deep down inside that she was not going anywhere without me. I kissed her on her cheek and said goodnight and told her I would be back first thing in the morning.

On Wednesday, November 14th I left home at 8:00 am and at the nursing home at 8:10 am. As I walked down the hallway towards Mom's room a since of urgency returned deep inside of me, again. I felt as if I was being pulled toward her room by some magnificent force greater then what I wanted to face. As I put my hand on the handle of her door to open it, I took a deep breath and asked God to please give me the strength that I knew I needed when I walked into her room. As I entered her room and saw her lying in bed I was totally caught off guard and all the strength that I had in those few seconds of entering her room completely disappeared. Her eyes were closed, her breathing much more labored, but yet there was this foam of saliva coming out of her mouth. My first reaction was that she was choking to death and it scared me. I felt so helpless for her and yet knew I needed to stay strong for her. I reached for the towel that was beside her bed on the nightstand and wiped her mouth gently. I kissed her cheek and with tears rolling down my eyes I called John on my cell phone and told him to come, to come as quickly as he could. Once again, I was afraid to be alone. I then left her room and went to the nurse station and cried to one of the nurses that Mom was actively dying. She told me she knew and returned to Mom's room with me. She was very compassionate and held me and hugged me until I gained composure. I knew I had to be strong for Mom. Within ten minutes John walked into the room and stood behind me with his hands on my shoulders as I sat beside Mom holding her hands, kissing her hands and praying out loud. I expressed my love for her and told her I knew she was walking with Danny and Dad and that they were leading her to heaven to be with God. I knew she heard me and through this whole time of kissing her hands and holding her hands and praying and talking to her she had her eyes closed. She then opened her eyes and I looked deep inside of them and told her I loved her so very, very much and that I would miss her and it was at this very moment she said "I love you". Just as she did, I felt deep within my soul her pulling me inside of her soul as if to take me with her. She exhaled one long breath and I said to John "she has passed" and his reply to me was "how do you know" and I said there should be one more exhale of breath and he bent down kissed her on her forehead and she exhaled the last breath. Mom passed at 8:38 a.m. that morning. "Dear God thank you for answering my prayers." I wasn't alone after all. "Dear God thank you for letting me be beside Mom, holding and kissing her hands." "Dear God thank you........Momma's last words spoken "I love you" were meant for me." I knew now that Dad was at true peace having her beside him and I too was at peace knowing they were reunited, after being only 36 days apart.

I had read only a few times in my lifetime of couples passing within a short span of each other. I never imagined that it would be my parents. Yet, after seeing it happen I only then realized the true love they had for each other. They came together 61 years ago and were only apart from one another for 36 days. God had a plan for them and I'm blessed that I was witness to a large part of his plan.

Epilogue

March of 2008, Mom and Dad were laid to rest at Arlington Cemetery in Washington, DC. Their family and friends joined together to pay their respect to a courageous soldier and father and a wonderful mother. God had blessed us with perfect weather that day. The night prior to their service I had received a phone call from the Chaplin who would be presiding over the service. He informed me that the service would be approximately thirty minutes long and his part of it would take approximately ten minutes. He asked me to share with him some stories about Dad and Mom. I thought to myself, how I could compress a life time of two wonderful people into just ten minutes. As soon as I felt overwhelmed and afraid that I would not do my parents justice, a peace subsided over me. It was God holding my hand. I shared with the Chaplin my father's diary from World War II. I shared with him many wonderful stories of Mom and Dad's life together. I was on the phone with him that night for over an hour.

The day of the service he did justice to the life of Mom and Dad. The Chaplin quoted with tears in his eyes the September 17, 1944 excerpt out of Dad's World War II Diary.

As the Chaplin quoted Dad's diary it was at this very moment I realized this was a true celebration of Dad's life. My father, the great man that he was and will always be in my heart was truly a magnificent man who was so full of joy, compassion and strength. Dad was with us that morning, because I felt him smiling and witnessed his light shining down on us.

He spoke kind and gentle words about Mom. Spoke of the incredible woman she was and will always be in my heart, as well as her joy for life and compassion for self and others. Mom was with us that morning, because I felt her smiling and witnessed her light shining down on us.

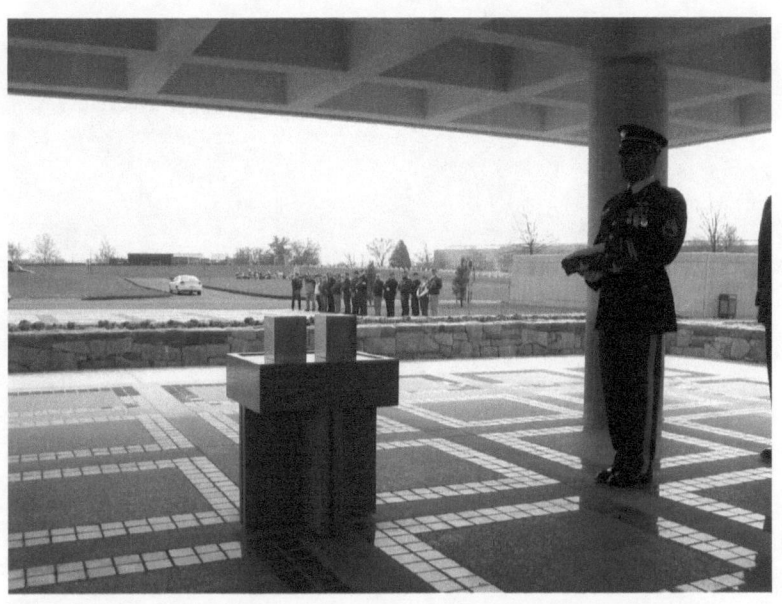

God saw they were getting tired
And a cure was not to be
So He put His arms around them
And whispered "come to Me."
With tearful eyes we watched them suffer
and saw them fade away
Although we loved them dearly
We could not make them stay.
Golden hearts stopped beating
Hardworking hands to rest
God broke our hearts to prove to us
He takes the very best.

Author Unknown

www.ingramcontent.com/pod-product-compliance
Lightning Source LLC
Chambersburg PA
CBHW031251280526
45784CB00004B/1802